The Mentality Of Humans

The Influence of Alcohol on Health, Family and
The Human Mind.

Nicholas Flamel.

1

Table of contents

Chapter One

Alcohol Itself

Alcohol has addictive qualities and is a toxic, psychoactive substance. It is a chemical that can be found in alcoholic beverages like wine, beer, and liquor. Additionally, it can be discovered in some medications, mouthwashes, home goods, and essential oils (scented liquid taken from certain plants). Alcoholic beverages are a common part of the social landscape for many people in many modern societies. This is especially true for people who frequent highly visible, globally influential social settings where drinking often goes hand in hand with socializing.

A drug is alcohol.

It is categorized as a depressant, which means that it slows down essential processes, causing slurred speech, shaky movement, foggy perceptions, and a slow response time.

The central nervous system is the target of its depressant action. This indicates that it reduces brain activity. Your mood, behavior, and self-control may change as a result. It may impair one's memory and ability to think clearly. Your physical control and coordination may be impacted by alcohol as well. When it comes to how it affects the mind, it's best to think of it as a substance that impairs one's capacity for reason and clouds their judgment.

Despite being a depressant, the type of effect depends on how much alcohol is consumed. The majority of drinkers do so to feel more energized, such as when they "loosen up" with a beer or glass of wine. But when someone consumes more alcohol than their body can handle, they start to feel depressed. They begin to feel foolish or have trouble controlling themselves.

An excessive intake of alcohol has even more potent depressive effects (inability to feel pain, toxicity where the body vomits the poison, and finally unconsciousness or, worse, coma or death from severe toxic overdose). How much and how quickly is consumed affects these reactions.

The Process
All alcoholic beverages, including wine, beer, and spirits, can be consumed.

How is booze produced?
The type of alcohol found in the alcoholic beverages we consume is a substance known as ethanol. The only type of alcohol used in beverages is ethanol (ethanol), which is created when grains and fruits are fermented. Alcohol is produced during the

chemical process of fermentation, which takes place when yeast interacts with specific food ingredients.

You must put grains, fruits, or vegetables through a process known as fermentation in order to make alcohol (when yeast or bacteria react with the sugars in food - the by-products are ethanol and carbon dioxide).

Describe fermentation.

Fruit is used to ferment to make wine and cider, while barley and rye are used to ferment cereals to make beer and spirits.

How long a beverage ferments has an impact on its alcohol content.

In a process known as distillation, a portion of the water from spirits is removed to leave a stronger concentration of alcohol and flavor.

There are various types of alcohol.

Different Alcohols

Anyone who has ever been to a grocery store is aware of the variety of alcohol available. Some types of alcohol are distilled, which increases their concentration of alcohol and makes them riskier.

Alcohol has been consumed by people for thousands of years, and it is now understood to be both a chemical and a psychoactive substance. When a hydroxyl group, which is made up of two oxygen and hydrogen atoms, replaces the hydrogen atom in a hydrocarbon, an alcohol is created. Secondary alcohols are produced when alcohols interact with other atoms. These secondary alcohols include methanol, isopropanol, and ethanol, the three types of alcohol that people regularly consume.

The Three Alcohol Types

Ethanol is the only form of alcohol that people can consume without risk. The other two types of alcohol are not used to make drinks; instead, we use them for manufacturing and cleaning. For instance, methanol (also known as methyl alcohol) is a component of boat and car fuel. Other products made with it include antifreeze, paint thinner, windshield wiper fluid, and many others. The chemical name for the rubbing alcohol we use for cleaning and disinfection is isopropanol (or isopropyl alcohol). Because our bodies metabolize methanol and isopropanol as toxic substances that result in liver failure, they are both poisonous to humans. Even a small amount of rubbing alcohol or methanol can be fatal to consume.

Over two billion people drink ethanol (also known as ethyl alcohol) every day. Yeast, sugars, and starches are fermented to create this kind of alcohol. People have been consuming ethanol-based beverages like beer and wine for centuries to alter their mood. Ethanol, however, also has negative effects on the body. Only a small amount of ethanol can be metabolized by the human liver.

Since ethanol is toxic, it gradually harms the liver, the brain, and other organs. Additionally, ethanol inhibits the central nervous system, which affects judgment and coordination. A person may also develop a crippling alcohol addiction as a result of binge drinking and other alcohol abuse behaviors.

Alcohol, Both Distilled And Undistilled

Distilled and undistilled alcoholic beverages fall into separate categories. Fermented drinks are another name for non-distilled beverages.
Both beer and wine are fermented, undistilled alcoholic drinks. While breweries ferment barley, wheat, and other grains to make beer, wineries ferment grapes to make wine.

The step after fermentation is distillation. A fermented substance becomes one with an even higher alcohol content thanks to the process. By removing it from the water and other ingredients of a fermented substance, distillation concentrates alcohol. Spirits and liquors are distilled alcoholic drinks. By volume, they have more alcohol than non-distilled beverages. An alcoholic beverage that has been distilled typically has a higher alcohol proof.

Measures of alcohol content, or the amount of alcohol in a drink, include alcohol by volume (ABV) and alcohol proof. Alcohol by volume is the amount of ethanol present in a solution expressed as milliliters per 100 milliliters (3.4 fl. oz.), whereas alcohol proof is the reciprocal of alcohol by volume. A beverage with a 50% ABV, for instance, will be 100 proof.
DRINKS CONTENT

Beer and wine are examples of fermented beverages that range in alcohol content from 2% to 20%. Alcohol content ranges from 40% to 50% or more in distilled beverages, or liquor.

For each, the typical alcohol content is:
Beer has an alcohol content of 2-6%.
Cider 4-6% alcohol
8–20% alcohol by volume in wine
40% tequila alcohol
40% or more alcohol in rum
40% or more alcohol is in brandy.
Gin contains 40–47% alcohol.
Whiskey contains 40–50% alcohol.
vodka with 40–50% alcohol
Alcohol content ranges from 15 to 60 percent in liqueurs.

Various Alcoholic Drinks Sorted by Alcohol Content
There are numerous varieties of alcoholic beverages, and some of them have higher alcohol content than others. Higher alcohol

content alcoholic beverages have the ability to quickly and in smaller doses lead to intoxication and alcohol poisoning.

Undistilled Beer is the most popular alcoholic beverage worldwide. In fact, beer is the most popular beverage consumed worldwide, followed by water and tea. The oldest alcoholic beverage in recorded history is most likely beer. Although some beers have higher or lower alcohol content, a typical beer, whether it be a lager or an ale, has an alcohol content of between 4% and 6%. For instance, "light beers" have an ABV of only 2% to 4%, whereas "malt liquors" have an ABV of 6% to 8%.

Wine
Another well-known and traditional alcoholic beverage is wine. The ABV of typical wine is less than 14%. The most popular sparkling wine, Champagne, has an alcohol content of 10% to 12%. In order to "fortify" some wines, distilled alcohol is

added. Fortified wines include, but are not limited to, Port, Madeira, Marsala, Vermouth, and Sherry. Typically, their ABV is around 20%.

Brut Cider
Apple juice fermented into hard cider. Typically, the ABV is around 5%.

Mead Mead has a 10% to 14% ABV and is made from fermented honey and water.

Saké Saké, a popular Japanese beverage made from fermented rice, has a roughly 16% ABV alcohol content.

distilled beverages (Liquors and Spirits)
Gin
Gin is a spirit that is typically created from a base grain like wheat or barley that is fermented before being distilled. However, the primary flavor of the beverage must be that of juniper berries in order for it to be recognized as gin; otherwise, it cannot bear

the name. Most gins range in alcohol by volume from 35% to 55%.

Brandy
Wine is distilled to make brandy. Brandy contains between 35% and 60% alcohol by volume. For instance, Cognac, a well-known brandy, has an ABV of 40%.

Whiskey
A spirit created from fermented grain is whiskey. Whiskey has an ABV that varies from 40% to 50%.

Rum
Rum, a distilled beverage made from fermented sugarcane or molasses, typically contains 40% alcohol by volume (ABV). Some rums are "overproof," which means they contain at least 57.5% ABV of alcohol. The majority of overproof rum is stronger than this requirement, typically reaching 75.5% ABV, or 151 proof.

Tequila

One kind of alcohol is tequila. The Mexican agave plant serves as the primary component of tequila. Tequila typically has an alcohol content of 40% ABV.

Vodka In the US, vodka typically has an alcohol content of 40% ABV and is made from fermented grains and potatoes.

Absinthe

Various leaves and herbs are used to create the alcoholic beverage absinthe. Absinthe does have a high alcohol content, but there is no proof that it is a hallucinogen. While some varieties of absinthe have an ABV of around 40%have as much as 90%.

Everclear

The grain-based spirit Everclear is another alcoholic beverage with a high alcohol content. Everclear has a minimum ABV of 60% but can also have a maximum ABV of 75.5% or 95%.

Chapter Two

Alcohol over the years

Numerous cultures and civilizations, including the Sumerians, Egyptians, Greeks, Romans, Chinese, and the British, have been impacted by alcohol throughout history. Alcohol consumption has both united and divided people throughout history, from the time that beer recipes were written down on tablets to Prohibition in the United States to the horrifyingly high rates of alcoholism in the present.

How old is alcohol, exactly?
Worldwide, fermented grains and fruits have been used to make alcohol for thousands of years. A lot of people are curious about the origins of alcohol, but there are many different theories. Remains in pottery jars dating from 7000 to 6600 B.C. in northern China are the earliest indication that people were brewing alcohol.

Sumerians

Beer was produced by Mesopotamian Sumerians between 3,000 and 2,000 B.C. On clay tablets, brew recipes for more than 20 different beers have been discovered. Because small grains of mash and grain remained in the unfiltered alcohol mixture, the Sumerians had to drink their beer through straws.

Research and ancient texts suggest that the Sumerians had laws and restrictions on alcohol use. But Sumerians also offered alcohol to the gods in sacrificial and religious ceremonies. An uncultured, underdeveloped man in the epic Sumerian tale Gilgamesh becomes one after consuming seven cups of beer.

Egyptians

Bread and beer were essential parts of the daily diet in ancient Egypt. Beer was revered as the nectar of the gods at the time. Usually made from barley, wheat, and yeasty dough, Egyptian beer.

The majority of Egyptians consumed beer due to its virtues and alleged nutritional advantages. Beer was recommended as a treatment for a number of ailments in an ancient medical text from this era. It served as labor compensation in Giza, where employees received three beer rations per day. At events and celebrations like the Tekh Festival, beer was also consumed (coined as The Festival of Drunkenness).

Greeks
One of the earliest known regions for wine production was Ancient Greece. Vineyards were first planted by winemakers in 2000 B.C. Early Greek religion placed a high value on alcohol, which was frequently offered to the gods. Additionally, it served as currency for the entire Mediterranean region.

Greeks and Egyptians both used alcohol as medicine. Greek texts frequently suggest drinking wine to treat medical conditions like lethargy, diarrhea, labor pains, and keeping wounds sterile and clean. Greek culture valued wine so highly that it even had its own deity, Dionysus. As the intermediary between the living and the dead, he was also revered as the god of fertility, ritual madness, and ecstasy.

Symposium, where affluent men would congregate to drink together, converse, tell tales and jokes, and engage in lively debates, was a popular event during this time. For each event, the wine strength was chosen by the symposium arch. Ancient Greek literature highlighted the connections between drinking and celebration, including Plato's Symposium, Homer's Iliad, and the Odyssey.

Romans

Greek winemaking was adopted by the Romans. The play Bacchae, which was written by a Greek poet, describes how the devotees of the god Bacchus indulged in excessive drinking and committed murder while high. The Roman Senate forbade the practice of Bacchic rites in Italy by 186 B.C. They thought that these followers might pose a risk to everyone's safety.

To increase local demand for Roman wine, the Roman Empire also imposed limitations on the development and harvest of grapevines. The Romans exported wines during the first two centuries B.C., frequently as payment for slave labor.

But after the anti-Bacchic purge, Roman attitudes toward drinking shifted. The military started to receive wine as a standard ration. The production of alcohol quickly became standardized, and the Romans produced bulk wine and model vineyards. Roman authors recommended wine and even berated people for drinking water. The fabled tale of Bacchus was adopted as their own, and the character was portrayed as a mythical but capable being with a humorous sidekick.

Chinese

China's relationship with alcohol has a complicated past. Ancient Chinese sources frequently mention drinking "natural alcohol." This organic alcohol is the result of fruit and floral natural fermentation.

Spirits made from bases that had undergone yeast fermentation were first distilled in China. Similar to other cultures, China also regarded alcohol as sacred. During significant rituals and occasions, like family gatherings, weddings, and holidays like the New Year, drinking was commonplace. Drinking went along with listening to music, dancing, and reading books.

The Chinese also held the notion that alcohol could treat and prevent diseases, lessen the effects of aging, and maintain general health. According to a traditional Chinese proverb, alcohol is the best medication.

All of these ancient cultures used alcohol for a variety of medical benefits, including the relief of headaches, the prevention of colds, the boosting of immune systems, the prevention of bowel problems, and the promotion of general health.

The 16th and 17th Centuries in British Alcohol History

The first overuse of distilled spirits in England occurred between 1525 and 1550. At the same time, experts talked about how common drunkenness is in England. The English made reference to drunkenness as a crime for the first time.

In 1600, during James I's reign, authors wrote about the widespread intoxication that pervaded all social classes. Almost every aspect of life included the use of alcohol. The Act to Repress the Odious and Loathsome Sin of Drunkenness was enacted by the English Parliament in 1606.

When Britain started taxing distilled spirits in 1643, the moonshine industry grew as a result. Gin was created in Holland around 1650. Soon after the drink was made available to British soldiers fighting in the area, the English gin industry began to expand. Soon after, in 1700, both Scotland and Ireland gained notoriety for their high-quality whiskies.

Native people experimented with their own alcohol recipes in other parts of the world, such as South America during the Inca era. Indigenous people in these areas used maize to make the chicha beverage.

American history of alcohol

The English were unfamiliar with drinking water when they first came to America and assumed that it was contaminated and unsafe, which it frequently was. They detested it because it was free and only ate it when they had no other options because they couldn't afford it. However, colonists started making their own beer in the 1630s using malted barley imported from England.

Massachusetts reaffirmed its anti-homebrewing laws in 1654. However, a law prohibiting the use of alcohol as payment led to a severe labor strike.

Colonial Americans drank throughout the day, favoring cider and beer, and eventually rum and the Founding Fathers were big drinkers. Americans started drinking rum in large quantities by the end of the 17th century because New England, where molasses was first distilled, soon had more than 140 distilleries. Alcohol consumption in America peaked in 1830 at 7.1 gallons per person, up from 5.8 gallons per person in 1790. (compared to 2.3 gallons today).

The Whiskey Tax of 1791 marked the culmination of these facts about alcohol history. As a result, Pennsylvania witnessed the Whiskey Rebellion, in which workers at distilleries protested and refused to pay the tax. Thomas Jefferson, the president, revoked the tax in 1802. The United States produced roughly 88 million gallons of alcohol annually in 1860, just before the Civil War.

In the 19th and 20th centuries, alcohol significantly impacted the Civil War. Chaplains used it in their ministries, as did nurses, doctors, and dentists for medication and sedation. Alcohol played a significant role in commemorating important occasions like the Fourth of July and New Year's Eve during the war.

However, because of the prevalence of abuse, many soldiers acted recklessly and dangerously while impaired. Alcohol was linked to rape and other violent war crimes.

Beginning in the early 1800s, the temperance movement gained momentum over the course of the following century. The initial goal was to cut back on alcohol consumption out of concern for the negative effects of binge drinking. As some people worked toward societal and personal reform, the movement served both religious and social objectives.

The half-pint rum ration for sailors was soon eliminated by the US Navy in 1862, and by the late 19th century, support for Prohibition (which outlawed the production and sale of alcohol) had grown. In 1919, it was changed to the 18th Amendment. Alcohol could only be produced or sold for medical or religious purposes, and it could only be consumed in one's home if it was purchased legally, according to the 1919 Volstead Act.

However, alcohol consumption itself was not prohibited during Prohibition. With the aid of organized crime and in speakeasies, many Americans bought and drank it. Many people thought that making alcohol legal would help the economy in the early 1930s, and in 1933 the 21st Amendment ended Prohibition.
Not long after, alcohol addiction treatment was developed.

Chapter Three

Alcoholism, its causes and prevalence.

What is alcoholism?
Alcoholism is a complicated, multifaceted phenomenon, and the many formal definitions of it change depending on who is defining it. According to a crude definition, alcoholism is a disease brought on by persistent, compulsive drinking. According to a purely pharmacological-physiological definition, alcoholism is classified as a drug addiction because it requires consuming increasingly larger doses to have the desired effects and because quitting drinking results in a withdrawal syndrome. However, this definition is flawed because, unlike other drug addicts, alcoholics do not always require ever-increasing alcohol doses. The increased amounts to which alcoholics become adapted are rarely above the normal single lethal dose, in contrast to opium addicts who become so accustomed to the

drug that they can survive more than a hundred times the usual lethal dose. Additionally, the withdrawal symptoms associated with alcoholism appear erratically, occasionally failing to manifest in someone who has already gone through them and never doing so in some drinkers whose destructive behavior is otherwise difficult to distinguish from that of a person who is pharmacologically dependent on alcohol.

According to a third, behavioral definition, alcoholism is a disorder in which alcohol takes on a prominent role in a person's life and in which that person loses control over how they want to use it. According to this definition, alcoholism may or may not be accompanied by physiological dependence, but it is invariably characterized by excessive alcohol consumption that results in repeated physical, mental, social, economic, or legal difficulties as well as regret. Due to the fact that such a behavioral disorder lasts for years, is strongly hereditary, and is a leading cause of death and disability, clinicians refer to it as a disease. Alcohol also permanently changes the brain's plasticity with regard to having the freedom to start or stop drinking episodes. Prospective studies show that willpower in and of itself has little predictive value, similar to other medical diseases but unlike the majority of bad habits.

Simply put, alcoholism is an alcohol addiction that results in abusing the toxic substance. It involves the misuse of drugs. Alcoholism is defined as the excessive and repeated consumption of alcoholic beverages to the point where the drinker repeatedly suffers harm or causes harm to others. The harm could be social, legal, economic, or physical or mental. Most clinicians, but not all, consider alcoholism to be an addiction and a disease because such use is typically thought to be compulsive and under noticeably diminished voluntary control.

what occurs after drinking alcohol.

It enters your bloodstream after being absorbed through your stomach's lining. Once there, it spreads throughout your body's tissues. In just five minutes, alcohol reaches your brain, and within ten minutes, it begins to have an impact.

Your liver begins processing alcohol after 20 minutes. The liver can metabolize one ounce of alcohol on average every hour. It takes roughly five and a half hours for a blood alcohol level of 0.08, the legal limit for drinking, to leave your system. Alcohol can linger in the body for up to three months in hair follicles and up to 80 hours in urine.

When you consume more alcohol than your body can effectively break down and metabolize, you become intoxicated.

Alcohol overdose symptoms include shaking, convulsions, vomiting, headaches, hallucinations, and convulsions.

It seems that the idea of chronic intoxication as a disease dates back to ancient times.

A knowledgeable minority view holds that the medicalization of alcoholism is incorrect, particularly among sociologists. The inability to control one's drinking does not occur constantly or in every circumstance, unlike most disease symptoms. The alcoholic is not always forced to drink; on occasion, they are able to fight the urge or drink in moderation. The early signs of alcoholism vary from culture to culture, and an uninformed observer may occasionally mistakenly label recreational public intoxication as alcoholism. The range of daily alcohol consumption in the general population is distributed along a smooth continuum. The medical model, which assumes that alcoholism is either present or absent—as is the case, for instance, with pregnancy or a brain tumor—contradicts this characteristic. For these reasons, according to the sociological definition, alcoholism is merely one sign of social deviance, and its diagnosis frequently depends on the perspective and moral framework of the observer. For instance, routine drinking can result in illness that requires days off from work. This makes alcoholism comparable to a disease in a contemporary industrial society. However, in a rural Andean society, occasional intoxication at designated communal fiestas that results in illness and a suspension of work for a few days is considered normal behavior. It should be noted that festival drinking is a decision and does not lead to regret. Alcoholism should frequently be anticipated to disappear with maturation, as is the case with many other signs of social deviation, if the sociological model were entirely accurate. But this doesn't happen.

Last but not least, epidemiologists require a definition of alcoholism that enables them to spot alcoholics in a population that might not be accessible for individual examination. They may use statistics on the amount and frequency of alcohol-related hospitalizations and community drinking, a formula based on the frequency of cirrhosis deaths in the population, or arrests for alcohol-related misbehavior to define alcoholism.

alcoholism's root causes

Many theories about the origins of alcoholism are based on the constrained viewpoints of experts in particular fields or professions. These theories cover a wide range of topics, including bad character, environmental contagion, economic hardship (or affluence), gloomy childhoods, preexisting depressive disorders, easy and affordable access to alcoholic beverages, and sociopathy. More sophisticated theories acknowledge that alcoholism is typically brought on by a combination of factors and take into account the complexity of the disorder.

Lifetime prospective studies have frequently demonstrated that certain theories of alcoholism were false because they conflated cause with association. For instance, current research suggests that growing up with alcoholic parents is associated with alcoholism but not the direct cause of it.

Similarly, alcoholism is linked to depression but typically not the cause of it (in men, at least), and it is linked to self-indulgence, poverty, and childhood neglect but not the cause. Once more, parental alcoholism frequently causes poverty and unhappiness in children; the same parental alcoholism also raises the risk of later alcoholism in such children, but for genetic rather than environmental reasons.

Studies on twins and adopted kids have supported the widespread assumption that alcoholism can run in families. Although not inevitable, this genetic component reflects that some people have a predisposition that makes them significantly more susceptible to alcoholism than other people. There is currently no proof that this predisposition is determined by a single gene. Instead, there are likely many genes, each with relatively minor individual effects, that influence the risk of becoming alcoholic. In fact, recent research indicates that a large portion of the genetic risk may not be related to neurological vulnerability but rather to an increased resistance to the unfavorable effects of excessive alcohol consumption. In accordance with this proof, a genetic flaw that prevents acetaldehyde from degrading has been discovered (a metabolic product of alcohol). Numerous individuals of Asian descent who are homozygous (carry two identical copies of the gene) for this defect experience a distinct and frequently unpleasant flushing reaction to even small amounts of alcohol, which lowers the likelihood that they will become alcoholics. Young women (but not young men) break down less alcohol in the stomach before it is absorbed through the digestive system due to another hereditary factor. Therefore, a given dose of alcohol results in higher blood alcohol levels in young women.

In addition to heredity, there are at least five other significant risk factors for alcoholism: peer pressure, cultural norms, some coexisting psychiatric disorders, accessibility, and employment.

The likelihood that someone will develop alcoholism is increased by peer social networks (friends, clubs, or spouses) that contain heavy drinkers and alcohol abusers. A well-mannered person might initially resist, but more often than not, such a person eventually gives in to peer pressure and participates. When this happens, the adage "if you can't beat them, join them" applies.

Additionally significant are social norms and cultural attitudes toward drinking. Low alcoholism rates are found in cultures where low-proof alcoholic beverages may be consumed with food or during religious ceremonies but where intoxication is taboo. High rates of alcoholism are found in cultures that tolerate heavy drinking but do not have traditions of drinking alcohol with food or in ritual settings. Alcoholism is more likely to occur in societies without any clear rules regarding alcohol consumption and societies where high-proof alcohol is consumed without food or ritual.

Alcoholism is also more likely in people who have certain psychiatric disorders, such as antisocial disorder, panic disorder, schizophrenia, and attention deficit disorder. Alcoholism is frequently used by patients with psychiatric conditions as a momentary escape.

The risk of alcoholism is also increased by ease of access.

Alcoholism is prevalent in areas or countries with low alcohol taxes, inexpensive alcohol that is heavily advertised, and little social control over alcohol sales. Finally, those who are unemployed, work jobs with unpredictable hours, like writers, or have long-term close contact with alcohol, like The development of alcoholism may be more likely in diplomats and bartenders.

For those who have abused alcohol for less than a year, a return to social drinking is frequently possible; however, if alcohol dependence has persisted for more than five years, attempts to resume social drinking typically result in relapse. The onset of chronic alcohol dependence for both men and women occurs most frequently from ages 25 to 50, despite the fact that the frequency of alcohol-related problems is highest among men aged 18 to 30. To put it another way, it frequently takes several years to develop into a chronic alcoholic with loss of control over the initiation and cessation of drinking. There are millions of young people who have the potential to become alcoholics through heavy drinking, but in many cases the process is not completed, and by the age of 30, many of these drinkers will have reverted to a pattern of social or voluntary drinking.

alcoholism is prevalent.
Depending on the definition used and the estimation techniques, estimates of the prevalence of alcoholism vary. Depending on how strict the criteria are, 10 to 20 percent of men and 5 to 10 percent of women in the United States will at some point in their lives meet the criteria for alcoholism. These rates are somewhat higher in eastern European nations but are comparable to rates for many western European nations. Rates are significantly lower in Southeast Asia and countries bordering the eastern Mediterranean. Rates in Africa are generally low, but in the newest urban slums, they are extremely high.

Comparing rates across nations is challenging, however, due to differences in the definition of alcoholism. Estimates of the prevalence of alcoholism have suggested rates that range from 1.1 to 11 percent in England and Wales and from 2.2 to 13 percent in Switzerland. Although more cautious estimates put the prevalence of alcoholism in France's adult population at 9 percent, higher estimates put it as high as 15%.

Despite having one of the highest per capita alcohol consumption rates in the world, Portugal did not even recognize alcoholism as a problem until the late 20th century. National per capita alcohol consumption is a significant factor in the prevalence of alcoholism. After the death of the Soviet dictator in the middle of the 20th century, there was an uproar that 40% of adult males in the Soviet Union were alcoholics, despite official denials to the contrary. However, statistics were insufficient in both cases. In summary, statistics on alcoholism contain a significant amount of subjectivity. Additionally, estimates of national consumption never consider whether illicit, untaxed alcoholic beverages are included, nor do comparative data consistently account for changes in diagnostic policies.

Chapter Four

Influence of Alcohol on the wellbeing (health)

What Are Alcohol's Effects on the Body?
Although you might not immediately feel the effects of alcohol on your body, they begin as soon as you take your first sip.

If you drink, you've probably experienced some of the effects of alcohol, from the warm buzz that starts to wear off quickly to the unpleasant wine headache or the hangover that appears the next day. You might not be overly concerned about them because they don't last long, especially if you don't drink frequently.

Many people believe that drinking a beer or a glass of wine once in a while at mealtimes or on special occasions is not particularly harmful. But consuming alcohol in any amount has the potential to have negative effects on your health.

Although those who binge or drink heavily may experience negative health effects more quickly, even those who consume alcohol in moderation face some risks.

What does it mean to consume alcohol moderately?
A moderate drinker is one who:

For women, one drink maximum per day.
For men, 2 drinks maximum per day.
A daily drink poses little risk of negative health effects, according to previous advice on alcohol consumption, and may even have some positive effects.

However, more recent research contends that there is actually no "safe" level of alcohol consumption because even moderate alcohol consumption can harm brain function.

Over time, alcohol use can start to negatively impact anyone's physical and mental health. If you regularly drink and have more than one or two drinks when you do, these effects might be more severe and obvious.

SUBTLE IMPACTS OF ALCOHOLS

Among the short-term effects you might experience while drinking alcohol (or right after) are:

feelings of drowsiness or relaxation

a feeling of joy or giddiness

Mood swings Lessened inhibitions

Impulsive actions

Speech that is slurred or slowed

nausea and diarrhoea

Diarrhoea

a headache

Hearing, vision, and perception modifications

Inability to coordinate

difficulty concentrating or making decisions

consciousness loss or memory lapses (often called a blackout)
After just one drink, some of these effects, like lowered inhibitions or a relaxed mood, might become apparent. After a few drinks, some additional symptoms, like loss of consciousness or slurred speech, may appear.

Effects of dehydration, such as nausea, headaches, and dizziness, can take a while to manifest and vary depending on what, how much, and whether you also drink water.

Even though these effects might not last long, they are still noteworthy. Impulsivity, lack of coordination, and mood swings can impair your judgment and behavior and have more severe consequences, such as contributing to mishaps, injuries, and decisions you'll later regret.

PERMANENT IMPACTS OF ALCOHOLS

Drinking alcohol can also result in longer-lasting issues that go beyond your own wellbeing and mood.

Regular alcohol consumption may have the following long-term effects:

persistent mood swings, including irritability and anxiety
Insomnia and other issues with sleeping
a weakened immune system, which could cause you to get sick more frequently
alterations in libido and sexual performance
Weight and calorie changes Memory and concentration issues
inability to concentrate on tasks
Conflict and tension in romantic and familial relationships have increased

THE PERSONAL IMPACTS OF ALCOHOL

The effects of alcohol on your internal organs and bodily functions are listed below.

DIGESTION AND ENDOCRINE SYSTEM

Over time, excessive alcohol consumption may result in pancreas inflammation and pancreatitis. Abdominal pain and digestive enzyme release can both be brought on by pancreatitis.

Serious complications and a long-term condition can result from pancreatitis.

LIVER DAMAGE

Alcohol is one of the harmful substances that your liver aids in the breakdown and elimination from your body.

Alcohol abuse over a long period of time impedes this process. Additionally, it raises your risk of developing chronic liver inflammation and liver disease brought on by alcohol:

A condition called alcohol-related liver disease can be fatal and cause your body to accumulate toxins and waste. Your liver may suffer long-term damage from scar tissue.

SUGAR LEVEL

Your body's response to glucose and use of insulin are both regulated by the pancreas. You may experience hypoglycemia, or low blood sugar, if your pancreas and liver aren't functioning properly because of pancreatitis or liver disease.

Additionally, a damaged pancreas may limit the amount of insulin your body can produce and use to use sugar. Hyperglycemia, or having too much sugar in the blood, can result from this. The complications and side effects of diabetes may worsen if your body is unable to control and balance your blood sugar levels.

If you have diabetes or hypoglycemia, experts advise staying away from excessive alcohol consumption.

CENTRAL NERVOUS SYSTEM

What is the most effective way to spot how alcohol affects your body? Recognize the effects on your central nervous system.

Alcohol impairs brain-body communication, which results in slurred speech, a crucial indicator of intoxication. Speech and coordination become more challenging as a result (think reaction time and balance). That is a key factor in the advice to never drive after drinking.

Alcohol can harm your central nervous system over time. Your hands and feet may start to feel tingly and numb.

Additionally, drinking can impair your capacity for

make lasting memories
Think clearly and make logical decisions
control your feelings
Drinking over time can also harm your frontal lobe, which is the area of the brain in charge of executive functions like abstract thought, judgment, social behavior, and performance.Wernicke-Korsakoff
syndrome, a memory-related brain disorder,

is one of the permanent brain injuries that can result from chronic heavy drinking.

DIGESTIVE SYSTEM
The link between drinking alcohol and digestive health may not be immediately obvious. Often, the side effects don't show up until after the damage has been done. Drinking more can make these symptoms worse.

Drinking can harm the tissues in your digestive tract, making it difficult for your intestines to properly digest food and assimilate vitamins and nutrients. Malnutrition may result from this damage over time.

Drinking excessively can result in:

Gas\sBloating
feeling of satiety in your stomach
diarrhea or uncomfortable stools

Infections or hemorrhoids (due to dehydration and constipation)
Without prompt diagnosis and treatment, internal bleeding brought on by ulcers may occasionally result in death.

CIRCULATORY SYSTEM
Drinking excessively over time can harm your heart and lungs and increase your risk of heart-related illnesses.

complications with the circulatory system include:
elevated blood pressure
abnormal heartbeat
blood pumping through the body is difficult.
Stroke
chest pain
Heart condition
heart attack
Fatigue can result from the body's inability to absorb vitamins and minerals from food;
Anaemia is a condition where your red blood cell count is abnormally low.

REPRODUCTIVE SYSTEM; Sexual and reproductive health
Alcohol will lower your inhibitions and enable you to perform tasks that would ordinarily be impossible.
However, excessive drinking can:

reduce the production of reproductive hormones
lower your libido make it difficult for you to achieve orgasm prevent you from obtaining or maintaining an erection
Drinking too much could alter your menstrual cycle and possibly raise your risk of infertility.

USE OF ALCOHOL WHILE PREGNANT
Alcohol consumption during pregnancy is not deemed safe at any level.

This is due to the fact that drinking while pregnant has effects other than on your health. It might result in a stillbirth, miscarriage, or early delivery.

After birth, newborns who were exposed to alcohol while still developing could develop a number of complications, such as:

learning challenges
persistent health problems
heightened emotional issues
development issues
muscular and skeletal systems
Alcohol abuse over a long period of time can reduce bone density, making bones brittle and raising the possibility of fractures in the event of a fall.
Bones that are weaker may also heal more slowly.

Alcohol consumption can also cause cramping, atrophy, and muscle weakness.

IMMUNE SYSTEM
Stemming from drinking a lot, Long-term heavy drinkers are also more likely than the

general population to contract tuberculosis or pneumonia. According to the World Health Organization (WHO), alcohol use is a factor in about 8.1% of tuberculosis cases worldwide.

Chapter Five

Diseases Associated with Alcoholism

Alcohol abusers have been shown to experience both acute and chronic illnesses to varying degrees. Worldwide, the risk of death from excessive alcohol consumption is higher than the risk of death from smoking, unsafe copulation, and illicit drug use combined. According to these figures, alcoholism is the most serious public health issue. Mortality is 2.5 times higher than expected among alcoholics. Alcoholism cuts life expectancy by 15 years, while heavy smoking cuts it by about 8 years. Up to 25% of patients in general hospitals in the United States are currently active alcoholics.

The severity of the social and psychological pathology linked to alcoholism is enormous, despite the fact that it is more difficult to quantify due in part to public denial. If uncounted, the number of patients hospitalized for personality disorders and depression brought on by alcoholism is significant. Parents who abuse alcohol greatly increase the likelihood that their kids will struggle in school, act out or use drugs.

acute ailments

Numerous changes to body chemistry, as well as neuromuscular, mental, and behavioral functions, are brought on by alcohol intoxication. Additionally, a drunk person is more likely to be involved in accidents and suffer injuries. According to studies, alcoholics who regularly experience severe intoxication are 30 times more likely to die from fatal poisoning, 16 times more likely to die from a fall, and 4.5 times more likely to die in a car accident. There is about a twofold increase in the risk of suicide, homicide, fire, and drowning. These liabilities are a reflection of both alcoholism-related poor self-care and the effects of immediate intoxication.

The acute alcohol withdrawal syndromes, which appear after intoxication, are additional acute conditions connected to alcoholism. The hangover, a general feeling of malaise frequently accompanied by headache and nausea, is the most frequent and least incapacitating of these syndromes. However, after a prolonged period of intoxication, severe withdrawal symptoms frequently take over. Trembling, loss of appetite, inability to retain food, sweating, restlessness, disturbed sleep, seizures, and abnormal changes in body chemistry are some of these symptoms (especially electrolyte balance).

Seizures, mental fogginess, disorientation, and hallucinations (both visual and auditory) are frequent symptoms of severe alcohol withdrawal. Delirium tremens may appear, typically after 36 hours, depending on the extent and caliber of care and treatment as well as the potential occurrence of additional disease. The symptoms of delirium tremens include fever, frank delirium, and a severe trembling of the entire body. If left untreated, it can last for three to ten days and has a reported mortality rate of five to twenty percent. Rarely, alcoholic hallucinosis that lasts for weeks to years can develop, with or without prior delirium tremens.

Wernicke disease, which results from an acute complete thiamin (vitamin B1) deficiency and is characterized by a clouding of consciousness and abnormal eye movements, may be brought on by prolonged drinking that prevents a healthy diet. Additionally, it may result in Korsakoff syndrome, which is characterized by an irreversible loss of recent memory and a propensity to compensate for the impairment through confabulation—the hasty recall of events without regard for the truth. Alcoholism and vitamin deficiency can also cause polyneuropathy, a degenerative condition of the peripheral nerves characterized by calf muscle tenderness, weakened tendon reflexes, and loss of vibratory sensation. Disorders of the gastrointestinal tract and liver inflammation and fatty infiltration are frequent (gastritis, duodenal ulcer, and, less often, severe pancreatitis). Cirrhosis, or chronic liver inflammation, can result in scarring.

Chronic conditions

The chronic disorders associated with alcoholism are psychological, social, and medical. Among the psychological disorders are depression, emotional instability, anxiety, impaired cognitive function, and, of course, compulsive self-deleterious use of alcohol. The mild cortical atrophy and impaired cognition that are frequently linked to alcoholism vanish after about six months of abstinence. There is typically noticeable improvement on tests evaluating chronic depression and anxiety after a highly variable period of abstinence, ranging from weeks to years.

Among the social disorders associated with alcoholism are 2- to 10-fold increases in driving and sexual offenses, petty crime, child and spousal abuse, and divorce. Homicide, homelessness, and chronic unemployment are several times more common among alcoholics than nonalcoholics.

Many of the chronic medical consequences of alcoholism are caused by dietary deficiencies. Alcohol provides large numbers of calories, but, like those from refined sugar, they are empty calories—that is, devoid of vitamins and other essential nutrients, including minerals and amino acids. The small amounts of vitamins and minerals present in beers and wines are insufficient for dietary needs. Alcoholics often skip meals during periods of heavy drinking or, due to digestive issues, are unable to absorb enough nutrients from their meals. Many of the chronic diseases connected to alcoholism are brought on by these nutritional deficiencies.

One or more of the chronic nutritional-deficit diseases may manifest in alcoholism with a long history. The more severe consequences of chronic thiamine deficiency—degeneration of the peripheral nerves (with potential permanent damage in severe cases) and beriberi heart disease—are probably the most frequent. Pellagra, which is brought on by a niacin deficiency, is another nutritional disease associated with alcoholism. Scurvy, caused by a vitamin C deficiency, hypochromic macrocytic anemia, brought on by a folate or vitamin B12 deficiency, or pernicious anemia, brought on by a vitamin B12 deficiency, are some of the other illnesses. Occasionally referred to as "wine sores," severe open sores on the skin of alcoholic recluses who typically consume cheap fortified wines are caused by a combination of multiple nutritional deficiencies and poor hygiene.

Cirrhosis of the liver (more specifically, Laennec's cirrhosis), which is frequently preceded by an organ enlargement caused by fat, is the disease that is most commonly linked to alcoholism. Alcohol-related cirrhosis is influenced by genetic susceptibility, the strain of metabolizing excessive amounts of alcohol, and poor nutrition. In its most severe form, Laennec's cirrhosis can be fatal; it is impossible to successfully treat cirrhosis or slow its progression in an alcoholic who cannot stop drinking. A person's risk of developing certain cancers, such as head and neck cancer (such as oral cancer and pharyngeal cancer), esophageal cancer, liver cancer, breast cancer, and colorectal cancer, is also increased by alcohol abuse. These conditions include fatty liver disease and alcoholic hepatitis.

In addition to the mental symptoms that may accompany pellagra, other mental disorders more specifically related to the consumption of alcohol include mild dementia, which may persist for up to six months after cessation of alcohol ingestion, and a relatively uncommon chronic brain disorder called Marchiafava-Bignami disease, which involves the degeneration of the corpus callosum, the tissue that connects the two hemispheres of the brain. Other brain damage occasionally reported in alcoholics includes cortical laminar sclerosis, cerebellar degeneration, and central pontine myelinolysis. Alcoholics, especially older ones, frequently experience enlargement of the ventricles as a result of atrophy of brain substance caused in part by the direct effects of alcohol on the central nervous system. In some cases, however, brain atrophy is the result of damage caused by accidents and blows. Many of those who survive long years of alcoholism show a generalized deterioration of the brain, muscles, endocrine system, and vital organs, giving an impression of premature old age.

Finally, chronic alcohol abuse heightens the risk of stroke and heart disease through cardiomyopathy, high blood pressure, and failed smoking cessation. It also greatly increases the risk of diabetes (by placing stress on the pancreas), of unwanted pregnancy and STD's (through unsafe practices), and of infection (by alcohol-induced suppression of the immune system).

Drinking alcohol can also factor your cancer risk:
Frequent drinking can increase your risk of developing:
Cancer of the mouth
Cancer of the throat
Cancer of the breast
Cancer of the oesophagus
Cancer of the colon
Cancer of the liver.

Drinking and using tobacco together can further increase your risk of developing mouth or throat cancer.

Chapter Six

Effects of Alcohol On The Brain.

Psychological effects

Long term alcohol intake can lead to a negative toll on the brain.

Concentration and recall
impulse management
Feelings, attitude, and personality
Regular drinking can have a negative impact on one's overall mental health and wellbeing, in part because it can make the symptoms of some mental health conditions, such as depression, anxiety, and bipolar disorder, worse.

With a hangover, you might also experience feelings of anxiety.

issues with mental health brought on by alcohol

When mental health symptoms closely resemble those of other mental health conditions, alcohol use can contribute to those symptoms.

The diagnostic criteria for the following conditions are contained in a mental health manual that mental health professionals use to identify mental health conditions:

drinking and bipolar disorder
psychotic disorder brought on by alcohol
insomnia brought on by alcohol
depression brought on by alcohol
anxiety disorder brought on by alcohol
You will only experience symptoms with these conditions during alcohol withdrawal or intoxication. Usually, these symptoms go away quickly after drinking is stopped.

Dependence
Some drinkers eventually build up a tolerance to it. They eventually have to drink

more in order to experience the same effects they once did.

Regular alcohol consumption can also result in dependence, which indicates that your body and brain are accustomed to the effects of alcohol.

You might experience a variety of physical, emotional, or mental health symptoms when you stop drinking, which go away as soon as you have a drink.

When your body becomes dependent on alcohol, you may experience tolerance and dependence as signs of alcohol use disorder, a condition that was formerly known as alcoholism. Depending on how many symptoms you experience, this condition can range from mild to severe.

Important signs might include:

Cravings

Withdrawal

Drinking more frequently over time and finding it difficult to stop after just one drink

drinking alcohol despite knowing that it affects your health or day-to-day functioning spending a lot of time on activities related to alcohol use

Your mind when drinking

Alcohol is absorbed throughout your entire body, but the brain is where it really suffers. The neural pathways in the brain are hampered by alcohol. Additionally, it may influence how your brain interprets information.

There are various levels of intoxication caused by alcohol:

subconscious intoxication

This is the initial stage of intoxication, with a blood alcohol content (BAC) of between

0.01 and 0.05. Although you may not appear to have consumed alcohol, your behavior, judgment, and reaction time may be a little off. Most men and women reach this stage after one drink, depending on weight.

Euphoria.

Your brain produces more dopamine when you first start drinking. This chemical and pleasure are related. You might experience euphoria and feel at ease and assured. Your memory and reasoning, however, might be slightly compromised. This stage, which is frequently referred to as "tipsy," happens when your BAC is between 0.03 and 0.12.

Excitement.

At this point, if your BAC is between 0.09 and 0.25, you are considered legally drunk. Your brain's occipital lobe, temporal lobe, and frontal lobe are all affected by this level of intoxication. Each lobe's function-specific side effects, such as blurred vision, slurred speech and hearing, and loss of control, can be brought on by excessive drinking. The processing of sensory data by the parietal lobe is also impacted. You might lose your fine motor skills and react more slowly. Mood swings, poor judgment, and even nausea or vomiting are common during this stage.

Confusion.

A BAC of 0.18 to 0.3 frequently resembles confusion. It affects your cerebellum, which aids in coordination. As a result, you might require assistance standing or walking. At this point, blackouts, or the brief loss of consciousness or memory, are also likely to happen. This is the result of the hippocampus, the part of the brain in charge of creating new memories, not functioning properly. Additionally, you might have a higher pain threshold, which could make you more vulnerable to injury.

Stupor.

When your BAC reaches 0.25, you might start to exhibit worrisome symptoms of alcohol poisoning. All cognitive, motor, and sensory processes are currently significantly compromised. There is a high potential for dizziness, suffocation, and injury.

Coma.

You run the risk of going into a coma at a BAC of 0.35. This happens as a result of impaired reflexes, motor responses, and breathing and blood circulation. A person in this stage is in danger of passing away.

Death.

A BAC of 0.45 or higher may result in death from alcohol poisoning or from the brain's inability to control essential bodily processes.

withdrawal from alcohol

Alcohol withdrawal can be challenging and, in some circumstances, fatal. If you want to stop drinking, you might need support from a healthcare provider depending on how much and how often you drink.

It is always advisable to speak with your doctor before stopping drinking. Going "cold turkey" might not always be a good idea.

Alcohol withdrawal symptoms include:

anxiety\nervousness
nausea\tremors
blood pressure is high.
unsteady heartbeat
heavy perspiration
Severe withdrawal can result in seizures, hallucinations, and delirium.

You can stop drinking in a healthy way with the aid of medical detox. Depending on your risk for withdrawal symptoms, your doctor may advise treatment at home or in a clinic.

Drinking guidelines
Although there isn't a completely risk-free way to drink, following these guidelines can help minimize some of the risks:

Don't forget to eat. To slow down the onset of intoxication, avoid drinking on an empty stomach.

Take in a lot of water. Make an effort to drink one glass of water for every standard beverage you consume.

Don't move too quickly. To give your body enough time to process the alcohol, sip slowly. One ounce of alcohol can be broken down by your liver each hour.

Avoid combining with other substances. Caffeine can mask alcohol's depressant effects, encouraging you to consume more alcohol than you otherwise might. You might feel more awake if you drink coffee to "sober up," but you might also be more likely to try to drive after drinking and make a mistake. Additionally, mixing alcohol and other drugs can be harmful.

Avoid drinking and driving. Don't ever drink and drive. You might still have alcohol in your system, which can slow down your reaction time, even if you feel like you've sobered up.

Chapter Seven

Mental health and Alcohol

Alcohol problems and mental ill health are closely linked. Alcoholism poisons the mentality and way of thinking of alcoholics and as such, leads to a series of problems related to mental health.

According to research, alcohol users are more likely to experience mental health issues. Additionally, it is true that those who suffer from severe mental illness are more susceptible to alcoholism. Alcohol can occasionally be used to treat the signs of stress, anxiety, and depression. Alcohol alters the communication between your brain cells, which can relax you.

They "self-medicate," or use alcohol to ease uncomfortable emotions or symptoms. Alcohol is sometimes used as a form of self-medication. While it may feel good at first, this effect is only temporary. The blissful feelings pass, and they may make your depression symptoms worse.

Your mental health may be suffering as a result of alcohol if:

a low mood, difficulty falling asleep after drinking, frequent hangovers, worry and anxiety in situations and around people you wouldn't normally worry about, and more are some severe effects of alcohol consumption.

after the feeling of calmness fades, mental health deteriorates
hangover symptoms such as headaches, nausea, and vomiting
anxiety and/or depression following alcohol use
Drinking excessive amounts of alcohol can exacerbate existing issues and make depression and anxiety worse over time.

The emergence of low self-esteem is one of the side effects of alcoholism that is frequently observed. The way we see ourselves is what is meant by having self-esteem. People who have high self-esteem frequently have positive opinions of themselves and exude confidence. People with low self-esteem, on the other hand, frequently have negative opinions of themselves and struggle to believe in their own abilities and worth.

People with alcohol use disorders frequently exhibit low self-esteem. Self-esteem may rise in the early stages of alcoholism, but as alcoholics become more and more isolated and lose contact with people who were once significant in their lives, it eventually tends to decline. Their optimistic mentality is destroyed by alcohol. Alcoholics may accept that they will always be addicted as a result of this decline in self-esteem, which may discourage them from seeking help. The following are some signs of low self-esteem:

the conviction that you are viewed negatively by others

Feeling like you can never succeed at anything Thinking poorly of yourself and believing others are out to get you

establishing or maintaining unhealthy relationships

having the impression that there is no way out of one's current situation.

depression and alcoholism

Depression symptoms have been linked to regular heavy drinking. When depressed people who drink alcohol stop, they frequently feel better within the first few weeks. If you give it a try and feel better, alcohol was probably the root of your depression. If your depressive symptoms persist, seek assistance from your doctor.

Drinking is generally not advised if you are taking antidepressants. Alcohol can worsen depression and make some antidepressants' side effects worse. According to research, some antidepressants may increase your risk of relapsing if you're trying to reduce or stop drinking.

anxiety and alcohol
If you have anxiety, alcohol may temporarily make you feel more at ease, but this feeling will pass. If you depend on alcohol to ease your anxiety, you might find that you need to drink more and more to unwind over time. This can eventually result in alcohol dependence.

A hangover may also make your anxiety worse.

If you drink to relax, consider other alternatives, such as meditation, yoga, exercise, or carving out time for your hobbies.

Alcohol and mental illness

If you regularly consume large amounts of alcohol or if you are a heavy drinker who abruptly stops drinking, you could develop psychosis.

Alcohol, self-harm, and suicide
Alcohol may cause you to act impulsively and lose control, which may result in behaviors like self-harm or suicide.
In this case, self-harm is used as a means of escape from the self-loathing that results from alcoholism. Self-harm is frequently used as a way to respond to and manage emotional pain, overwhelming feelings, or distress.

Most of the time, people who self-harm do not intend to end their lives, but this is not always the case. Some people discover that self-harming causes physical pain, which temporarily dulls the emotional pain.
Suicidal ideas and attempts are also associated with heavy drinking.

Chapter Eight

Alcoholism and its effects on Family

Alcoholism is frequently described as a family disease. Although it does tend to run in families, this is not the reason alcoholism is referred to as a family disease. This is due to the fact that one person's alcoholism has an impact on the entire family.

Within a family, alcohol abuse and alcohol use disorder, which is the medical term for an alcohol addiction, can cause strife or even lead to the dissolution of the marriage. As a result, those who abuse alcohol run up huge debts, start arguments, neglect their kids, and generally harm the wellbeing of the people they care about. Family members may eventually start to exhibit codependency symptoms, unintentionally maintaining the addiction despite the harm it causes. Rehab and family therapy are beneficial.

Some effects of problem drinking on loved ones, coworkers, employers, co-students, and others include the following:

Neglect of important responsibilities: Alcohol impairment impairs one's cognitive and physical abilities, which eventually will probably lead to neglect of obligations related to work, home life, and/or school.

Alcohol has a number of immediate side effects, including the need for time to recover from hangovers. Although the physical effects of a hangover may pass quickly, they can seriously impair a person's capacity to fulfill obligations and encourage unhealthy habits like poor eating and inactivity.

Legal issues: Drinking can make it more likely for someone to get into fights, act disorderly in public, drive while intoxicated, or engage in domestic violence or other violent behavior.

Alcohol is an addictive substance that can result in physical dependence, which is the inability to stop using it at will. Continuous drinking is a slippery slope that can lead to addiction, even though a person who is physically dependent (i.e., has an increased tolerance among other side effects) is not necessarily addicted.

In essence, alcohol abuse leads a person to prioritize drinking.

The time, energy, and resources that were previously devoted to life-sustaining activities, like working and spending time with family, are disrupted as a result.

At first, a person may believe that drinking alcohol helps them cope with these stressors, but regular heavy drinking can eventually lead to dependence on the drug. Alcohol abuse can take over a person's life once they develop a psychological addiction to it. It is simple to understand how alcohol abuse affects a person's entire network of family, friends, coworkers, employers, and anyone else who depends on them because people are frequently a part of social networks.

Parental Issues

Parents who abuse alcohol may become irrational and unstable. As the illness worsens, they become less capable of being parents. Alcoholics frequently behave inconsistently around kids, which gives them confusing messages. One instance of conflicting messages could be the acceptable consumption of alcohol, which raises the possibility of underage drinking.

Developing Children

Academic difficulties are more common in children of alcoholic parents than in children without such parents. A child's ability to function emotionally and develop psychological disorders may be hampered by divorce and parental anxiety brought on by a family history of alcoholism. Adult children of alcoholics may exhibit impulsivity, difficulty forming close friendships, or excessive dishonesty.

Alcohol Abuse Leading to Domestic Abuse. Alcoholism can exacerbate relationship issues, including money problems and child care concerns. Communication that is emotionally abusive can result from any of these factors.

The following categories of emotional abuse can result from alcoholism:

Using insulting or demeaning language
Threats of physical violence
Embarrassing behaviors or words
intimidating remarks or behaviors
manipulating or blackmailing
Alcoholism and intimate partner violence are linked, in addition to emotional abuse.

According to the World Health Organization, some studies indicate that drinking alcohol worsens both the frequency and seriousness of domestic violence. Alcohol abuse may be a risk factor for domestic violence or its cause.

Alcohol does, however, obviously impair critical thinking abilities and self-control. These negative effects prevent good, productive communication that can be used to settle disputes.

Alcoholism and financial difficulties

Alcohol costs money. Even the most strict accountant or budgeter can allow for entertainment costs, but frequent drinking can quickly push people to go over their budget for socializing. It is well known that abusing alcohol can cause serious financial issues, but not just because of the money used to buy alcohol.

Alcohol may lower your inhibitions, making it more likely for you to make impulsive purchases without considering the long-term effects of those decisions. For instance, a drunk person might be more likely to overspend at the bar than they had intended. Even drinking at home does not protect you from overspending when your guard is down. The internet provides access to a vast array of shopping options. The "beer goggles" effect can increase the likelihood of an unnecessary purchase by making an item seem more appealing and the purchase price seem more inviting.

Alcohol abuse can reduce productivity at work. Finances encompass potential earnings in addition to actual earnings. Drinking has been linked to decreased work or academic performance across the board, according to studies. College students who binge drink may have lower grades, which may have an impact on other students, their employment prospects and salary potential.

Absenteeism is more likely in workers who binge drink or drink heavily.

Binge drinking raises healthcare costs by $249 billion annually and reduces worker productivity. Numerous factors, including: Alcohol abuse can increase debt, particularly credit card debt.

a decline in income from work making it difficult to pay off credit card debt.
increased credit card charges to close the income and expense gap.
charges related to drinking or drinking-related behaviors, such as partying or gambling.
forgetfulness regarding the due date for payments, leading to late fees and other consequences.
Chronic drinkers may also need to quit their jobs early due to health issues.

Numerous health problems, including cirrhosis, pancreatitis, pneumonia, cardiovascular diseases, and various cancers, are linked to heavy drinking.

Social Security and employer-sponsored or independent retirement account contributions are reduced by a decrease in earned income. Additionally, if a health insurance plan had been partially funded by an employer, a loss of employment may result in higher out-of-pocket expenses.

Families need a specific amount of income to cover their expenses. The difference between expected earnings and expenses and actual earnings and expenses can widen when a person starts abusing alcohol. Because of this, the person's personal stability (if they are single) or family life may be severely disrupted.

Alcohol and Relationship Issues
Whether the drinker is a parent, child, member of the extended family, or an older adult like a grandparent, alcohol abuse is a

significant source of stress within a family. Due to the special dependence that spouses have on one another, the other is likely to experience the negative effects of one spouse's alcohol abuse. By law, spouses are considered to be a single financial entity (though this is not always the case; for instance, one spouse is typically not responsible for the other spouse's student loan debt). Drinking can exacerbate issues and jeopardize a relationship when it drains finances and/or results in health problems. The most frequent issues that arise between spouses when one partner abuses alcohol include the following, according to the National Institute on Alcohol Abuse and Alcoholism:

Marital strife.
Infidelity.
Domestic abuse.
unanticipated pregnancy
economic instability
Stress.

Jealousy.

Divorce.

Financial instability can easily lead to serious issues in a marriage, as was discussed earlier in relation to the actual and potential economic losses brought on by alcohol abuse and debt. An extensive range of emotions, including those related to abandonment, unworthiness, guilt, and self-blame, can be brought on by a spouse's alcohol abuse. All of these feelings may come together to form codependency, a disorder.

People may become maladjusted to a loved one's drinking, leading them to facilitate it by providing care. Alcohol abusers often have physical problems that necessitate other people's assistance. While some people might be able to control their urge to lend a hand, many people won't, especially partners, kids, and other family members or concerned people in the person's immediate vicinity.

Alcohol abuse has torn apart many families and friendships, and those who have experienced such tragedies typically experience trauma, mental retardation, and cognitive impairment.
The effects of alcohol on the family are what will ultimately have an impact on society.

In other words, alcohol has no beneficial effects on people's mentality.

Chapter Nine

Curbing Alcoholism

You must first comprehend your relationship with drinking in order to stop consuming beer or any other alcoholic beverage. From there, you might require ongoing self-care, social support, and new routines that can help you change your perspective.

The social aspect of drinking is widely accepted, as is its use as a stress reliever. It might even be a treatment for anxiety or insomnia.

However, drinking generally does little to alleviate these worries over the long term. There are also some significant drawbacks.

As a result, you might consider whether a break is necessary. You're not alone either. Numerous initiatives, such as month-long sobriety challenges and the #The SoberCurious movement, are encouraging people to examine their relationship with alcohol.

These suggestions can assist you whether you're looking to cut back or take a permanent break.

1. Examine the health effects of alcohol
There are many ways that alcohol can harm your health. Even a small amount of alcohol can make you feel sleepy, disoriented, or hungover. Drinking more increases your likelihood of noticing additional negative health effects, such as:

disturbed slumber

intestinal problems

memory issues

Anxiety, depression, and irritability are all on the rise.

disagreements and other disputes with family members

These effects may start to compound over time.

2. Investigate your relationship with alcohol over a period of time.

Knowing why you're doing something is a crucial first step in giving it up.

Determine how much you actually consume. Even if you don't believe you are dependent on alcohol specifically, you may still be concerned that you may be.

Say that when you abstain from drinking, you don't experience any cravings. But "a quick drink" frequently turns into three or four. When you're having fun, it's difficult to stop, especially when you're with friends who are also enjoying themselves.

Consider your drinking habits and your alcohol triggers.
It's possible that your worries are more about why you drink than how much. Many people turn to alcohol to dull their emotions or cope with stressful situations better. It's common to drink to ease tension before a challenging conversation or a first date.

But if you find it difficult to deal with problems without alcohol, you might want to think about whether drinking keeps you from developing more effective coping mechanisms for your emotions.

Knowing the causes of your drinking can help you look into more effective solutions to those problems. among typical alcohol triggers are:

stress in relationships social gatherings working problems and insomnia
You can make plans to help manage the urge to drink by becoming more aware of your alcohol triggers and motivations.

3. Think about your strategy
You might be aware of your desire to completely stop drinking. However, you might be unsure of quitting entirely and unwilling to hold yourself to that objective.

That's totally acceptable. The most crucial thing is to examine your drinking patterns and find a way to reduce it that works for you.

Without complete abstinence, it is still possible to improve one's relationship with alcohol and make more thoughtful, knowledgeable drinking decisions.

Prudence management
One option to complete sobriety is moderation management.
It puts an emphasis on finding the best strategy for your situation, not someone else's, with a view to reducing alcohol use and the potential harms that come along with it.
Of course, achieving total sobriety isn't a bad goal, but it doesn't have to be the only one.

Not yet certain of your end goal? That's also okay. Just be aware of your options.

4. Discuss it

Sharing your decision to stop drinking with others may inspire you to stick with your resolution.

Include your family.
When you stop drinking, your family and friends can encourage you and support you. Sharing your experiences with alcohol could inspire others to examine their own drinking patterns.

Perhaps your spouse, sibling, or roommate is contemplating a change as well. Together, you can support each other while increasing your motivation and accountability by quitting drinking.
You should keep in mind how crucial it is to go to events with alcohol with a trusted support person. When you're not by yourself, it's frequently simpler to decline a drink.

Find a neighborhood

Developing new connections with people who refrain from drinking can be very advantageous. The more assistance you receive, the better.

Here are a few concepts:

Why not invite a different coworker to check out the brand-new bakery down the street instead of putting your resolve to the test by going to the usual happy hour with your colleagues?

Think about developing relationships with people who don't view alcohol consumption as a high priority in their lives.

Miss the ambiance of the bar? You might be able to go to a sober bar and mingle without drinking depending on where you live.

Knowing what to say

People may query you as to why you decline a drink. You're not required to provide specifics, but it can be useful to be prepared with the following response:

"I'm reducing my spending for my health."
I dislike how drinking makes me feel.
Having said that, all you need to say is "No, thanks." You can feel more at ease and assured when you find yourself in an alcohol-related situation by practicing your refusal beforehand.

Since the majority of people are unlikely to notice or remember what you do, try not to worry about how they might perceive you. Keep your explanation straightforward if you want to give loved ones a more thorough explanation but are unsure of what to say: "I've been drinking a lot without a clear reason, and I want to spend some time rethinking that habit."

"I catch myself drinking when I don't want to face my emotions, and I want to get better at working through them without alcohol."
"I don't really enjoy drinking, and I'm tired of doing it just because everyone else does."

5. Modify your surroundings
Drinking can become a sort of automatic reaction when alcohol is a regular part of your routine, especially when you're stressed or overwhelmed.

Making a few adjustments to your environment to help prevent alcohol triggers can have a significant impact on your ability to stop drinking. You may not need to completely reinvent your life in order to succeed.

Throw away your alcohol.
When you're trying to quit, having alcohol around your home may tempt you. Knowing you'll need to go out and make a purchase

can dissuade you from having a drink long enough to find a suitable diversion.

Have non-alcoholic drinks on hand for both you and other people. Being a good host doesn't require you to serve alcohol. Allow visitors to bring their own alcohol, and allow them to take it with them when they depart.

If you share a home with roommates, think about suggesting that they keep their alcohol hidden rather than in common areas.

Discover a new favored NON-ALCOHOLIC beverage.
Making the right substitution beverage choice can support you in remaining steadfast in your decision to stop drinking. Even though plain water has many health advantages, it's not the most exciting option.

You can find something enjoyable to do without missing your favorite beverage if you put a little creativity into it.

Try adding cinnamon sticks or other spices to tea, apple cider, or hot chocolate, or infusing plain or sparkling water with chopped fruit or herbs. You can also combine juice or lemonade with sparkling water.

Change up your routine to stay busy.
One of the best ways to break a pattern of drinking at a particular time of day is to divert your attention to something else. The most beneficial activities are those that regularly get you outside and moving.

If you can't resist temptation, steer clear of locations that sell alcohol.
Consider taking a walk or meeting your friends for a hangout in the park or another alcohol-free area if you typically meet up with friends for drinks after work.

Why not try a new place that doesn't serve alcohol instead of going to your usual restaurant for dinner and drinks? You'll have the opportunity to do something unusual without being tempted to drink.

To pass the time and save money, make it a habit to cook at home.

Having a few different coping mechanisms available can help when your desire to drink is more influenced by your mood than any particular time of day:

Try affirmations, deep breathing exercises, or meditation as alternatives to drinking to reduce anxiety.

Reach out to a loved one or watch a favorite movie to make yourself feel better when you're feeling lonely.

6. Get ready for a possible alcohol detox

When they significantly reduce or stop drinking, people who are more dependent on alcohol may begin to experience what is known as alcohol detox. As your body starts to flush alcohol from your system, this occurs. Alcohol withdrawal symptoms, such as: can be brought on by detox.

anxiety\headache\fatigue
insomnia
Mood swings cause sweating
If you're worried you might experience withdrawal symptoms when you stop drinking or cut back, speak with a healthcare provider. You can devise a strategy to get through it together.

7. Schedule self-care time
Giving up alcohol can be very stressful. Alcohol can be used to treat emotional distress, but the additional stress can increase the urge to drink, making success seem even more improbable.

Making significant changes can be challenging, but good self-care habits can help you deal with overwhelming emotions and look after your body and mind.

Prioritize your health

Being physically at your best can increase resiliency and emotional fortitude, enabling you to withstand situations that make you want to drink.

You're taking a big step toward bettering your physical health by abstaining from alcohol. You'll probably feel more energised and motivated to continue your progress as you start to experience those health benefits.

Additional pointers:

Remain hydrated.
Frequently consume balanced meals. Include foods that give you more energy and improve your mood.
If you can, engage in regular physical activity.
Prioritize getting more rest. Most adults should aim for 7 to 9 hours per night.
rekindle passions

Alcohol is a common way for people to deal with boredom. In addition to helping you relax, which is something everyone needs to do, satisfying hobbies can divert your attention from the desire to drink.

The time is now to pursue an old hobby if you've recently discovered that you miss it.

Even when you are unable to physically engage in activities with others, technology makes it simpler than ever to learn new skills and develop unique connections.

You could try:

maintaining a journal
Though journaling may not have ever piqued your interest, it can be a useful tool for tracking your emotions as you attempt to give up alcohol.

You may be able to identify patterns that provide more understanding into your alcohol use by exploring in writing what you find challenging and when you feel the most like drinking.

You can identify times when drinking doesn't help with the issues you're attempting to manage by contrasting the emotions that arise when you drink with the emotions that arise when you refrain from doing so.

A journal also provides a helpful place to list your motivations for quitting and come up with alternatives to drinking.

You can vent to a loved one or work on improving your communication to rekindle your relationship when you want to drink to avoid conflict or stress in your relationship. You might look into ways to connect with far-away friends or consider finding new friendships if loneliness makes you want to drink.

Self-compassion is ultimately one of the most crucial resources you have at your disposal.

Remember that no one is perfect, so don't be hard on yourself if you're having a hard time or if you slip up and have a drink. Your capacity to keep an open, inquisitive mind as you discover what works and doesn't for you is what matters most.

Know your Motives.
Along the way, you might encounter challenges that tempt you to drink. Remember the factors that led you to reduce or stop drinking. If you want a physical reminder to look at when you need it to help motivate you to stick with it, consider writing them down and keeping notes on hand.

9. Request assistance.

There's no need to go it alone; some people find it harder than others to stop drinking on their own.

Consider seeking out professional assistance if you're having trouble sticking to your goal or simply need more direction.

Talk to your primary healthcare provider about your difficulties if you feel comfortable doing so. If you feel awkward talking to your doctor, looking for a therapist can be a great place to start.

Additionally, you can get assistance from detoxification facilities.
a hospital stay.
Outpatient therapy
behavioral medicine.
mutual-aid organizations

Giving up alcohol can take some time. If it initially doesn't stick, be kind to yourself. Whether your ultimate goal is total abstinence or just more moderate drinking, you're still doing your body and brain a lot of good.

Chapter Ten

Turning Down and letting go of Alcohol.

Have excuses
Stick with soda
Nurse a drink
Talk with the bartender
Be honest
Offer to drive
Be firm in your refusal
Change the subject

Alcohol is a significant component of the social scene in many communities. Alcohol is frequently consumed at events like college parties, weddings, and informal get-togethers with friends.

However, what if you don't drink?

You might be recovering or you might just be taking a break to see how it goes. In either case, you want to avoid drinking any alcohol during the evening.

It can be awkward to decline alcohol, especially if you're with people who have witnessed your drinking in the past.

These advice can help you get through the situation, whether you've made the decision to abstain from alcohol permanently or you're just having a night off.

Prepare some justifications.
You can always be up front about the reasons you don't drink, but you shouldn't feel pressured to.

Telling a small white lie to get your friends off your back is not harmful. Perhaps it is technically accurate, but that isn't why you don't drink. It's a straightforward way to decline drinks in either case.

Here are a few possible justifications:

You have an early class or shift at work, you're still groggy from the previous night, and you're meeting your family for breakfast at a ripe hour.
Telling someone you're taking an antibiotic or another medication that interacts poorly with alcohol may stop them from interrogating you. People won't typically challenge you about your health.

Choose a non-alcoholic beverage.
You could bring sodas or any other non-alcoholic beverages of your choice if

you're meeting friends outside. You're less likely to be offered a drink if you're already holding one, which helps you avoid some potentially awkward interactions.

If you plan to go out to a bar, many of them offer alcoholic-free beers and ciders. If you'd prefer, there are also always other options, such as soda, juice, or water.

Put on a fake drink.
The advice below is somewhat similar to this, but it might be more effective for you.

You can "nurse" a drink by pouring it out in the bathroom or giving it to friends to try if you feel comfortable holding alcohol without actually drinking it.

Perhaps you don't mind a little alcohol, but you don't want to get wasted. You could place an early-evening drink order and gradually sip on it throughout the night, leading your friends to believe you ordered several drinks.

Consult the bartender
A quick chat with the bartender won't harm you if you want to appear to be drinking. The majority of them won't treat you differently because you don't drink alcohol, and they serve everyone.

For instance, if you order a coke, you can request that it be served in the same glass as a vodka coke. There won't be any suspicion because the two drinks appear to be identical.

You can go one step further with cocktails and order one that doesn't contain alcohol but ask the bartender to set it up and decorate it to look like it does. The worst thing they could say is "no," which is improbable.

Be truthful

In the short term, justifications might work. However, you might think about telling the truth if you're with reliable friends or if you're planning on abstaining from alcohol for a while.

It's acceptable to be open about your decision to abstain from alcohol since everyone has a different relationship with it. Being honest can keep your friends off your back over the long term, as opposed to making up justifications that might only work up until the next time you go out with them.

Who knows, you might even learn that someone else is coping with a comparable circumstance.

Request a ride
Why not volunteer to be the designated driver since everyone should be aware of the dangers associated with drinking and driving?

Your friends will appreciate you for sticking together, and you can enjoy your time out without worrying about drinking.

To refuse, be adamant.
Whether it's the truth or an excuse, you don't have to give anyone an explanation.

It's acceptable to simply say "no" to someone if you don't feel like explaining yourself. You have the right to keep your business private, especially if the other person is a stranger.

You might discover that people aren't bothered, though. Sometimes it's harder to resist drinking in a social setting than it actually is. People frequently just don't care.

Additionally, if there is limited alcohol available at a party or other event, you are doing everyone a favor by leaving more for the other guests.

After all, you're just saying no for yourself and not trying to regulate their drinking habits.

Changing the topic

They might inquire as to why if they notice you aren't drinking. Alcohol has a way of lowering people's inhibitions, so even if they are a friend who is aware that you don't drink, they might still inquire or press for more information.

You can change the topic if you don't feel like responding, especially to a drunk person. Ask them about themselves, for instance, or engage them in conversation about something unrelated to alcohol.

The Synopsis
There are various reasons people choose not to drink, and it is entirely up to you to decide how transparent you want to be about your own situation.

Just keep in mind that choosing to drink or not depends on you. Even if you're the only one not drinking, you can still have fun with your friends as long as everyone is understanding of one another's preferences.

A common strategy for quitting drinking is to reach the proverbial "rock bottom" and then look for help from peer support groups or physical treatment facilities. At least, that's how many people used to view alcohol use disorder recovery. But in modern times, you don't have to go broke or declare yourself a "alcoholic" to rethink whether your relationship with alcohol is benefiting your life.

People are starting to understand that abstaining from alcohol for a while can have advantages thanks to the recent popularity of 30-day challenges like Dry January and Sober October. However, if you're new to sober curiosity, you might be unsure of how to start considering your relationship with alcohol.

It need not be a frightening or intimidating process. Think to yourself, "maybe I should check in with myself about my alcohol consumption," just as you might think, "maybe I should get more sleep this week." Here's a starting point.

To start, ask yourself if alcohol is still beneficial to you.
Even if you don't see alcohol as a major issue in your life, periodically evaluating your relationship with alcohol is a wise move.

Is alcohol preventing you from living your life or doing the things you want to do? It can be beneficial to consider how alcohol affects the four main areas of your life, which include:

The state of my mind

physically healthy
Relationships
daily activities and work
Consider what transpires while drinking and the day after to see if alcohol is having a negative effect on your health, relationships, work, school, or mental health:

Do you argue more with friends and family when you're intoxicated?
Are you unable to take advantage of a beautiful day outside due to a hangover?
Does the amount of alcohol you drank the night before affect how productive you are at work or school?

If you're trying to stop drinking, it's crucial to identify what you were drinking to cope with (for example, drinking in social situations because you have social anxiety) and to find other coping mechanisms.

Keep in mind that drinking was a coping mechanism you used when something was stressful for you. Although this will be advantageous in the long run, it might hurt in the short run. I would advise allowing yourself the freedom to try new things and discover what works for you.

limiting your social interactions to only those you truly care about locating some enjoyable reading (more on this in a moment)
picking up a new hobby
Exercising
Breathwork and meditation
locating calming aromas
beginning work with a coach or therapist
In general, I'd advise you to treat yourself with kindness and compassion as your body and mind get used to a life without alcohol.

Create a network of allies
Your friends and family might not support you when you start to reevaluate your relationship with alcohol, especially if some

of them are the people you used to drink with.

Setting boundaries with the people in your life who still drink is crucial because sometimes those same people may feel judged by your evolving attitude toward alcohol. Since this is ultimately your life and your choice, consider setting boundaries, honoring your recovery goals, and prioritizing your needs."

In the early stages of sobriety, you can start setting boundaries by putting some distance between yourself and heavy drinkers. You can also look for others who are in the same situation as you.

I suggest connecting with sober people on social media if you're having trouble finding support systems as you experiment with quitting drinking or are unsure of how to make sober friends.

On social media, there are countless incredible accounts and quick challenges you can complete. There are numerous challenges, ranging in length from 30 days to a year. These are useful in understanding the effects of alcohol on the brain and in learning how to rewire our neural pathways with empathy for ourselves.

Following hashtags can help you find friends who are sober on social media.

Look into resources and read some literature
You can start reading quit literature if you think you might have a more severe case of alcohol use, also known medically as alcohol use disorder.

However, "quit lit" is a great place to delve into if you are soberly curious and want to explore your relationship with alcohol and some of the impacts that alcohol is having on your body and mind. There are many books in this relatively new category of self-help literature written by people who have stopped drinking or cut back. The genre of "quit lit" is limitless.

Recognize when seeking professional assistance to quit
If you've tried to reduce your alcohol consumption but were unsuccessful, you may require expert assistance to stop drinking.

It's crucial to get professional assistance if your efforts to reduce or stop drinking alcohol are unsuccessful.

It's also critical to pay attention to how your emotions change when you stop drinking. When you stop drinking, any difficult or uncomfortable feelings that you were coping with by drinking will likely get worse. To address and overcome these challenges, it is crucial to seek professional assistance in these situations.

This may be crucial if you struggle to stop smoking and experience withdrawal symptoms.

Alcohol withdrawal is serious, so if you suspect that you might experience severe withdrawal symptoms, I would recommend speaking with a professional before trying to stop drinking. If you are concerned that your body is becoming too accustomed to this substance, you should see a doctor or professional who specializes in addiction, such as a therapist.

But how can you tell if you might require expert's assistance? It is recommended talking with a healthcare professional if you notice you need to drink increasingly large quantities of alcohol to get the same effects you used to or if you notice withdrawal symptoms.

Even if you don't experience these symptoms and just want some extra help, it's worth reaching out. If you find that you are trying to stop repeatedly without success, getting professional help from a therapist or outpatient program may give you the best chance of wide-reaching recovery.

Above all, be gentle with yourself
Although, compared with other substances, there's less stigma for those who are on the spectrum of alcohol use disorder or even just sober curious, shame surrounding alcohol and quitting drinking is still very much real. In fact, it is found that shame was the second most common reason for people not seeking help, after lack of problem awareness.

Shame can be a real factor since traditional recovery programs rely on the label "alcoholic," which while helpful to those who prefer it can actually feel stigmatizing to those dealing with problem drinking as well as those just beginning to explore sobriety.

It's important to remember that labelling yourself is not necessary to take a step back and reconsider alcohol's role in your life. That's why it is recommended that you be kind to yourself and thinking about this as an experiment.

Remember that quitting drinking can be hard, so set realistic expectations for yourself. Remember to celebrate small wins, like your first night out without alcohol or telling a close friend about your decision to try sobriety or cut back on drinking.

Finding joy in sobriety by trying new things, moving your body, and planning alternate activities around the times you are most likely to want to drink, that way, you will negate the temptations.

And remember," 'No' is a complete sentence."

It is better to have never drunk, than trying to stop drinking because Habits are difficult to break.